WALL PILATES

Workouts for Women

30 DAY CHALLENGE

Improve posture, flexibility, muscle tone & heart health

HAZA ENZA

Wall Pilates is a great way to exercise at home or on the road — it's a low-cost, low-impact, highly effective way to increase your fitness level, stability, and flexibility without stressing your joints. Follow the instructions closely and refer to the illustration included with each exercise to ensure that your posture and technique is as good as it can be, and don't be afraid to use the included modifications to avoid straining or overstretching your muscles. Consistency is key, so you'll get the best results with daily practice. Good luck — and welcome to the new you!

Printed in the United States of America
Paperback ISBN: 978-1-961624-77-1

DartFrog Blue is the traditional publishing imprint of DartFrog Books, LLC.

301 S. McDowell St.
Suite 125-1625
Charlotte, NC 28204

www.DartFrogBooks.com

All you need is a wall and a commitment to daily exercise. You got this.

CHALLENGE DAY

1

ROLL UP AND ROLL DOWN

1.1 STANDING ROLL UP AND ROLL DOWN

How: Stand against the wall upright. Without moving your upper back, walk your feet one step away from the wall. Ensure that the back of your head, upper back, and mid back remain against the wall, and keep the hips neutral. Engage your core. Lift your arms as you inhale. As you exhale, engage into your deep core muscles to slowly peel away from the wall, vertebrae by vertebrae, and roll yourself down slowly to reach the floor. Take a moment here to breathe before rolling back up in your exhale, vertebrae by vertebrae, touching the wall with your hips, then your mid back, upper back, and the back of your head. Lastly, reach your arms overhead against the wall.

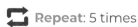 **Repeat**: 5 times

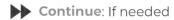 **Continue**: If needed

Modification: Keep a slight bend in your knees if your hamstrings are feeling tight.

Important notes: Keep a microbend in your knees and don't lock them.

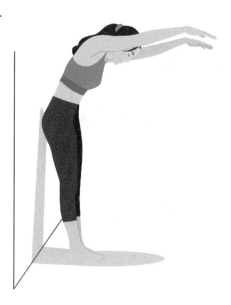

1.2 SEATED ROLL UP AND ROLL DOWN

How: Lower yourself to the floor with your back against the wall. Extend both legs straight out and next to each other, keeping your hips neutral. Your back should be flat on the wall with both sit bones grounded. Inhale and lift both arms, then slowly roll forward, vertebrae by vertebrae. Create a C-curve spine, peeling the back of your head away from the wall, followed by your upper back, mid-back, and lower back. Reach your fingertips to your legs or toes. Take a moment here to breathe before slowly reversing the motion and rolling back up to sitting, vertebrae by vertebrae, in your exhale until your back is against the wall.

 Repeat: 5 times   **Continue**: If needed

Modification: Keep a slight bend in your knees if your hamstrings are feeling tight. If your lower back feels uncomfortable, place a block or pillow under your hips for support.

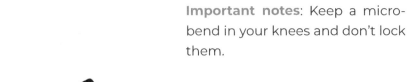

Important notes: Keep a microbend in your knees and don't lock them.

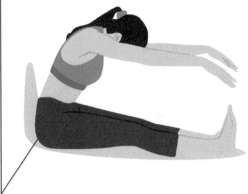

1.3 SEATED ROLL DOWN WITH OBLIQUES TWIST

How: Stay seated sideways against the wall with both legs extended next to each other. Ensure that both sit bones are grounded on the floor. Bring your arms forward as if you're hugging a tree. As you roll halfway back, vertebrae by vertebrae, turn towards the wall to work on the oblique muscle that is closest to the wall. Bring your palms to the wall for support. Slowly come back to center with your arms forward as if you are hugging a tree. Roll up slowly, vertebrae by vertebrae, until your spine is straight and you are upright.

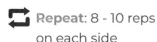 **Repeat**: 8 - 10 reps on each side

▶▶ **Continue**: 1 - 2 sets

Modification: Keep a slight bend in your knees if your hamstrings are feeling tight.

Important notes: Contract the oblique muscle that you are working on for maximum effect.

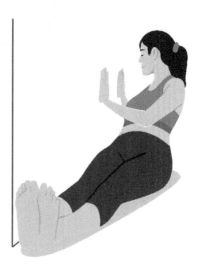

CHALLENGE DAY 2

2

STANDING PUSH-UPS

2.1   HIGH PLANK PUSH-UPS

How: Stand facing a wall at arms' distance from it. Place your palms flat against the wall at shoulder height. Spread your fingertips wide. Inhale as you lift your heels off the ground and lengthen your spine. Move your chest closer to the wall, keeping your elbows bent and your arms activated and close to your body. Stay for 3-5 breaths. Exhale and push away from the wall by straightening your arms, keeping your body straight and the back of your head, shoulders, hips, and heels aligned.

 Repeat: 5-10 times as you progress

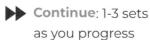 **Continue**: 1-3 sets as you progress

Modification: If you find keeping your elbows in challenging, you can widen your elbows while keeping them parallel.

Important notes: Maintain proper alignment, engage your core muscles, and keep your elbows close to your body.

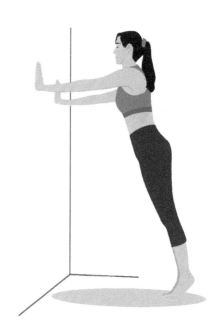

2.2 ELBOW PLANK PUSH-UP

How: Similar to exercise 2.1, begin with the elbows, forearms, and palms against the wall, with the elbows underneath your shoulder level. Push away from the wall by straightening the arms, keeping your palms flat against the wall. Lower down slowly as you bring the elbows back to the wall.

 Repeat: 10 reps   **Continue**: 3 sets

Modification: If you find it challenging to push from the elbows to straight arms, try just keeping the elbows off the wall as you push away, and then lowering them back to the wall in a controlled movement.

Important notes: Maintain proper alignment and engage your core muscles.

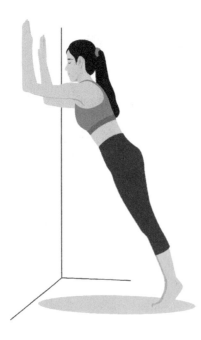

2.3   SINGLE ELBOW PLANK PUSH-UPS

How: Similar to exercise 2.2, but instead of placing both elbows against the wall, only place one elbow against the wall. Keep the other arm bent at the elbow and behind your back. Push away from the wall with a slow and controlled movement, maintaining the same chest level and height, then slowly return to your starting position.

 Repeat: 10 on each side   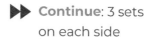 **Continue**: 3 sets on each side

Modification: Instead of placing the other arm behind your back, you can hold the arm sideways and keep the palm against the wall for support. If you find it challenging to push from the elbow to the straight arm position, try just keeping your elbow off the wall when you push out, and lowering the elbow back onto the wall with control.

Important notes: Maintain proper alignment and engage your core muscles.

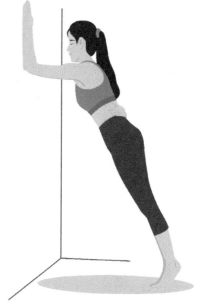

CHALLENGE DAY

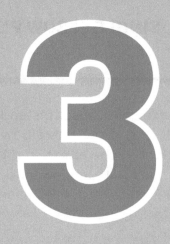

3

DRAW
THE
CIRCLE

3.1 USING THE FINGERTIPS

How: Stand next to the wall with one shoulder touching the wall. Inhale, lifting the arm next to the wall overhead. Keep the fingertips facing forward as you reach your hand above the shoulder, flip your palm to face away from the wall, exhale, and externally rotate your shoulders. Lower the hand to the side of your hip. Repeat 10 times before switching sides.

For internal rotation, flip the palm of the extended arm to face the wall. Inhale, and move the arm in a reverse circular motion until you reach the hip in exhale. Complete 10 rotations, then switch sides.

 Repeat: 10 external rotations & 10 internal rotations on each side

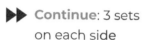 **Continue**: 3 sets on each side

Modification: Work the shoulder rotations within your range of motion.

Important notes: Your hip and chest do not rotate during these movements.

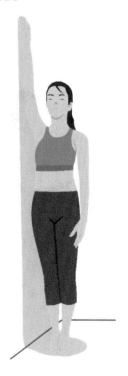

3.2   USING THE KNEE

How: Stand in front of a wall about 1-2 steps away from it. Bend one knee and keep it touching the wall. Point your toes. Try to balance here by bringing your hands to your hips and maintaining core engagement. Keep your gaze at eye level. Activate your glutes and slowly lead the edge of your knee to form a circle in an external rotation. Return to center. Complete 10 rotations.

For internal rotations, repeat the starting position above and move the knee in the opposite direction.

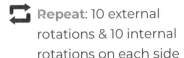 **Repeat**: 10 external rotations & 10 internal rotations on each side

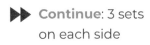 **Continue**: 3 sets on each side

Modification: Move slightly closer and bring your fingertips to the wall for additional support.

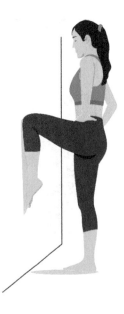

Important notes: Keep the chest and hips facing forward and avoid rotating them.

3.3 USING POINTED TOES

How: Stand in front of the wall at a distance of your extended leg. Bring your hands to your hips. Inhale, lift one leg, and point the toes to touch the wall. Engage the core and activate the glutes. Use your leg muscles to make a circle with your toes in a clockwise direction. Return to the center. Repeat 10 times before switching sides.

For internal rotation, begin in the same position as above. Make the circle with the toes in the opposite direction. Complete 10 rotations before switching sides.

 Repeat: 10 external rotations & 10 internal rotations on each side

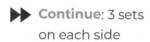 **Continue**: 3 sets on each side

Modification: Move slightly closer to the wall and bring your fingertips to the wall for additional support. You may bend your knee if you have hamstring limitations.

Important notes: Keep the chest and hips facing forward and avoid rotating them.

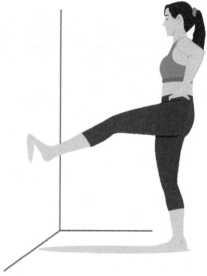

CHALLENGE DAY

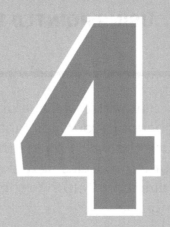

4

STANDING AIRPLANE

(palms on the wall)

4.1 SINGLE LEG (SIDEWAYS)

How: Stand facing the wall and walk about 2-3 steps back from it. Lightly touch the fingertips to the wall for balance. Lift one leg, engage the glutes, and activate the leg by flexing or pointing the toes and kicking sideways. Slowly return to the center.

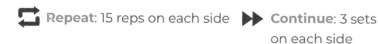 **Repeat**: 15 reps on each side ▶▶ **Continue**: 3 sets on each side

Modification: Kick sideways at a height that is comfortable for your range of motion.

Important notes: Continue looking forward at the wall while kicking sideways.

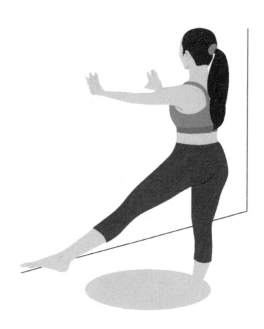

4.2   SINGLE-LEG (BACKWARD) EXTERNAL AND INTERNAL ROTATIONS

How: Similar to exercise 4.1, but instead of kicking sideways, kick backwards and hold the position with flexed or pointed toes. Externally rotate the leg for 10 reps, then internally rotate the leg for 10 reps, before returning to the original position.

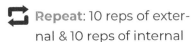 **Repeat**: 10 reps of external & 10 reps of internal rotations on each side

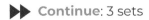 **Continue**: 3 sets

Modification: You may bend the knees if you have hamstring limitations.

Important notes: Continue facing the wall and ensure that hips face forward.

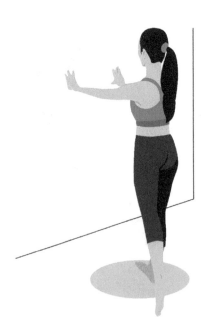

4.3 SINGLE BENT KNEE TO BACK LEG EXTENSION

How: Similar to exercise 4.1, but instead of kicking sideways, bend the knee facing the wall and kick backwards. Extend the leg with a flexed foot before returning to the original position. Repeat for 20 reps before switching sides.

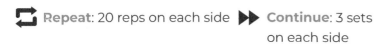 **Repeat**: 20 reps on each side 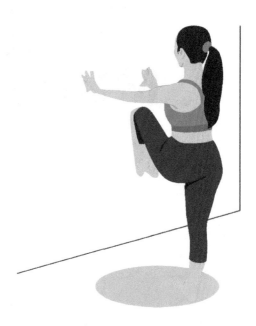 **Continue**: 3 sets on each side

Modification: Kick backwards according to your comfortable range of motion.

Important notes: Maintain core engagement to avoid overcurving the lumbar during the kickback.

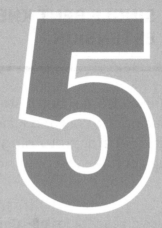

CHALLENGE DAY

5

ARM
MOVEMENTS

5.1 TWIST SIDE TO SIDE (MILD TWIST)

How: Stand about 2 steps away from a wall with your back to it. Lift your palms and bend your elbows. Keep your feet about hip distance apart. Start with your hips neutral. Inhale, look forward, exhale, and turn to one side for your spinal twist, pressing both palms against the wall before switching sides.

 Repeat: 10 reps   **Continue**: Up to 3 sets

> **Modification**: If you are unable to place both palms against the wall during the twist, focus on the spinal twist instead.

> **Important notes**: Spinal twist rotation should be initiated from the spine, not the hips.

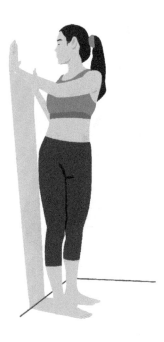

5.2 CACTUS ARMS IN CHAIR POSE HOLD

How: Stand about 2 steps away from the wall with your back to it. To make cactus arms, lift your palms and bend your elbows to 90 degrees. Place your cactus arms, the back of your head, your shoulders, and the back of your hips against the wall. Drop your hips to the same level as your knees at a 90-degree angle. Keep the feet together and your hips neutral. Engage your core and hold your chair pose while moving your cactus arms in extension upwards, and in flexion back down to shoulder height.

 Repeat: 15 reps   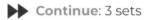 **Continue**: 3 sets

Modification: If you find there's a limitation in placing your elbows and knuckles against the wall, gently lift them away from the wall according to your range of motion.

Important notes: Be mindful of your knee joints here, and don't bend the knees beyond your toes.

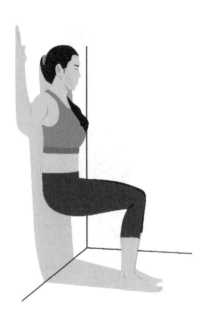

5.3   SNOW ANGEL ARMS IN LEG EXTENSION TO WIDE SQUAT

How: Stand about 2 steps away from the wall with your back to it. To make snow angel arms, lift your arms upwards and extend them out to the side while leaning onto the wall. Keep the palms touching the wall and your shoulders in internal rotation. Place the back of your head, your shoulders, and the back of your hips against the wall. To perform the wide squat, drop your hips to the same level as your knees, making 90-degree angles with the toes pointing outwards. When you're in your squat, your snow angel arms come down next to your hips. As you extend the legs to push back up to your starting position, your snow angel arms come up, as well. Continue with this flow for 30 reps.

 Repeat: 30 reps   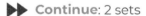 **Continue**: 2 sets

Modification: Instead of Snow Angel arms, you may just extend your arms to the side and move them up and down.

Important notes: Keep the legs active at all times by pressing your feet firmly on the ground.

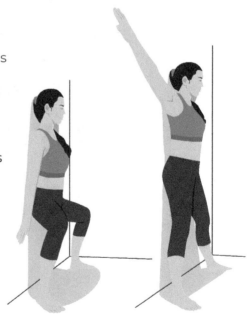

CHALLENGE DAY

6

SHOULDER RETRACTION AND PROTRACTION

6.1   STANDING FACING THE WALL

How: Stand facing the wall at an arm's length away. Place your palms against the wall, with your feet about hip distance apart. Engage your core and exhale to slowly protract your shoulder blades, moving them away from your spine. Inhale, drop your chest, and squeeze your shoulder blades to retract your shoulder blades towards the spine. Continue this flow for 20 reps.

 Repeat: 20 reps   **Continue**: 1-3 sets

Modification: None.

Important notes: Movements should be initiated from the shoulder blades. Keep your head, shoulders, and hips aligned.

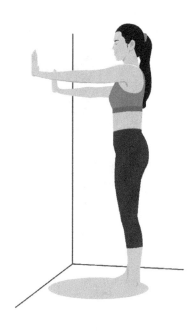

6.2 SHOULDER PROTRACTION IN STANDING HIGH PLANK WITH KNEE PULSES

How: Similar to exercise 6.1, but remain in shoulder protraction. Lift one knee and pulse forward continuously for 20 reps on each side.

 Repeat: 20 reps on each side ▶▶ **Continue**: 3 sets on each side

Modification: Lift the knee to pulse height according to your range of motion.

Important notes: Core remains engaged.

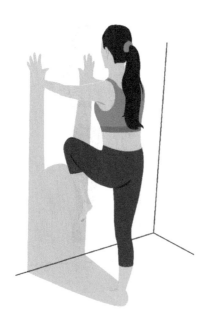

6.3
SHOULDER PROTRACTION IN STANDING ELBOW PLANK WITH ALTERNATE KNEE CRISS-CROSS

How: Similar to exercise 6.1, maintain shoulder protraction and come into elbow plank against the wall. Lift one knee to the opposite side of the body and switch continuously for 30 reps.

 Repeat: 30 reps   **Continue**: 3-5 sets

Modification: Lift the knee to a height that is comfortable for your range of motion.

Important notes: Core remains engaged.

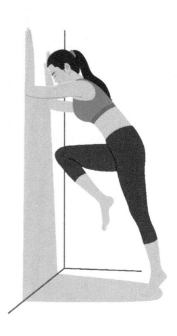

CHALLENGE DAY

7

STANDING STRETCH

7.1 LATS STRETCH

How: Stand sideways to the wall, about 1-2 steps away. With the arm nearest the wall, walk the fingertips up the wall to lengthen that side of your lats, then slowly drop the hip closest to the wall to stretch the lats. Lengthen this side for 30 seconds. Slowly push the palm against the wall to push the hip away from the wall. Lift the opposite arm to reach over the wall. Now use the palm closest to the wall to push away from the wall to assist and lengthen the opposite side of the lats. Stay here another 30 seconds.

 Repeat: 3 reps on each side 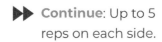 **Continue**: Up to 5 reps on each side.

Modification: Control the intensity of the stretch as you go.

Important notes:
Lengthen the lats slowly and with control for a gradual stretch.

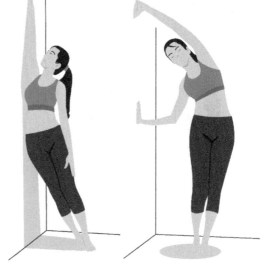

7.2 PECS & HAMSTRINGS STRETCH

How: Stand facing the wall with the feet about hip distance or wider apart as you go deeper in the stretch. Place your palms against the wall and walk backwards as you slowly lower your head between your arms. Open your arms to a V shape and lower your shoulders and hips to the same height to feel a good stretch. Stay here for 30 seconds.

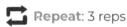 **Repeat**: 3 reps   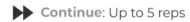 **Continue**: Up to 5 reps

Modification: Bend your knees if there are limitations on the hamstrings.

Important notes: Relax the head down and ensure there is no tension on the back of your neck.

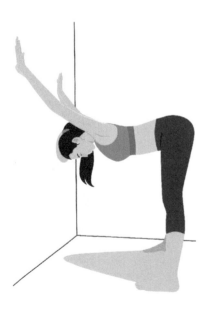

7.3   ARM & PECS STRETCH

How: Stand facing the wall with feet about hip distance apart. Place one palm on the wall, with the wrist slightly higher than your shoulder. Turn your torso in the opposite direction of the palm on the wall. Do not move the palm away from the wall during this turning movement.

Stay here for 30 seconds. Return slowly to center with your palm still on the wall before switching sides.

 Repeat: 2 reps on each side   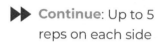 **Continue**: Up to 5 reps on each side

Modification: Instead of a straight arm, you can bend the elbow and forearm against the wall.

Important notes: Don't move the palm on the wall while turning. Keep the fingertips wide.

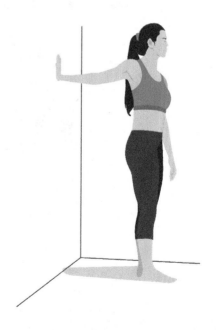

CHALLENGE DAY

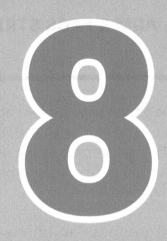

STANDING HIGH PLANK

8.1 HIGH PLANK ALTERNATE KNEE CRISS-CROSS

How: Stand in front of the wall with the palms on the wall about shoulder width apart. Keep the arms straight with a micro bend on your elbows and walk 2-3 steps back from the wall to achieve a good incline space from the wall. Protract your shoulder blades and engage your core. Lift your heels off the ground and bring one bent knee across the body to the other side. Then switch sides.

 Repeat: 30 reps   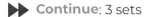 **Continue**: 3 sets

Modification: Keep the stabilizing foot flat instead of raising the heel.

Important notes: Maintain core engagement to avoid overcurving the lumbar, and keep the shoulder blades in protraction.

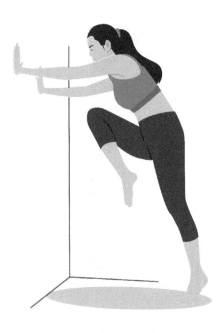

8.2   HIGH PLANK KICKBACK PULSES

How: Similar to exercise 8.1, but instead of a bent knee, lift one leg to kick back in pulses with a flexed or pointed foot. Engage the glutes to assist total core engagement.

 Repeat: 30 rep on each side   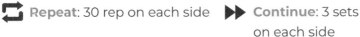 **Continue**: 3 sets on each side

> **Modification**: Keep the stabilizing foot flat instead of raising the heel. Kick back at a lower height.

> **Important notes**: Maintain core engagement to avoid overcurving the lumbar, keep the shoulder blades in protraction, and activate the glutes to avoid lower back discomfort.

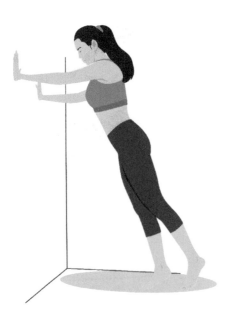

8.3 HIGH PLANK SINGLE RAINBOW TOE TAPS

How: Similar to exercise 8.1, but instead of a bent knee, lift one leg, point or flex that foot, and bring it across and over the back of the other leg.

 Repeat: 30 rep on each side   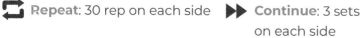 **Continue**: 3 sets on each side

Modification: Keep the stabilizing foot flat instead of raising the heel. Gently tap on the top of the opposite heel instead of crossing over the opposite leg.

Important notes: Maintain core engagement to avoid overcurving the lumbar, keep shoulder blades in protraction, and activate the glutes to avoid lower back discomfort.

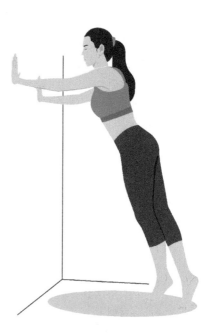

CHALLENGE DAY

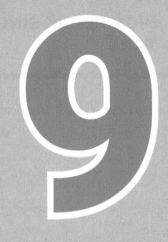

9

HIP
LIFTS

9.1 HIP LIFTS WITH A STRAIGHT BACK

How: Lie down on the floor and bring your hips close to the wall. Bend your knees and place your feet on the wall hip distance apart. Ensure that the knee and foot angle is 90 degrees, with your palms on the floor next to your hips. Press your palms down firmly and engage your glutes, inner thighs, and core as you push through your upper back to lift your hips, keeping the hips neutral. Stay here for 3 counts before lowering down gently.

 Repeat: 10 reps   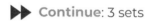 **Continue**: 3 sets

Modification: Adjust the height of the feet on the wall and lower the hips if necessary.

Important notes: Maintain the hips in neutral and avoid excessive curving of the lumbar. There shouldn't be any pressure behind the neck.

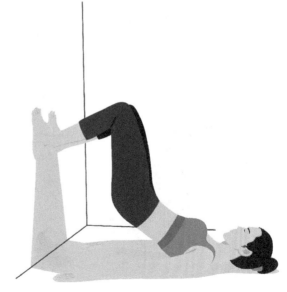

9.2 HIP LIFTS VERTEBRAE BY VERTEBRAE

How: Similar to the exercise above, but instead of a straight back, articulate your spinal movement by moving vertebrae by vertebrae.

Lie down on the floor and bring your hips close to the wall, bending your knees and placing your feet on the wall hip distance apart. Ensure the angle of the knees is 90 degrees and your palms are on the floor next to your hips. Press your palms down firmly and engage your glutes, inner thigh, and core as you push through your upper back and then tuck your tailbone to peel your lower back and mid-back away from the ground. Keep the hips neutral. Stay here for 3 counts before lowering down gently, first tucking your tailbone, then slowly landing on the floor with your mid back first, lower back second, and your hips last.

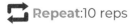 **Repeat**:10 reps   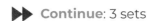 **Continue**: 3 sets

Modification: Adjust the height of the feet on the wall and lower the hips, if necessary.

Important notes: Try your best to articulate the spine movement. Maintain neutral hips and avoid excessive curving of the lumbar. There shouldn't be any pressure behind the neck.

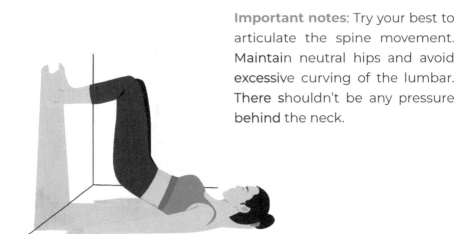

9.3   HIP LIFT PULSES

How: Adjust your position to exercise 9.1. As you get back down halfway, pulse your hips upwards.

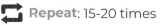 **Repeat**: 15-20 times   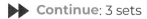 **Continue**: 3 sets

Modification: Adjust the height of the feet on the wall and lower the hips, if necessary.

Important notes: Do not put any pressure behind the neck. Press through the upper back. During the hip pulses, maintain both of the hips at the same height.

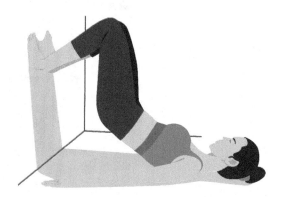

CHALLENGE DAY

10

HIP LIFTS WITH SINGLE LEG LIFT

10.1 SINGLE LEG LIFT UPWARD PULSES

How: Prepare your position for a hip lift exercise. As you lift your hips, hold this position and lift one leg straight upwards. Point your toes on the extended single leg. As you stabilize, start pulsing the single leg upwards.

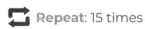 **Repeat**: 15 times

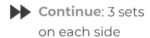 **Continue**: 3 sets on each side

Modification: You may bend the knee on the pulsing leg instead of the straight leg if there are hamstring limitations.

Important notes: Keep the hips at the same height during pulsing and lower down slowly to avoid any impact on your back.

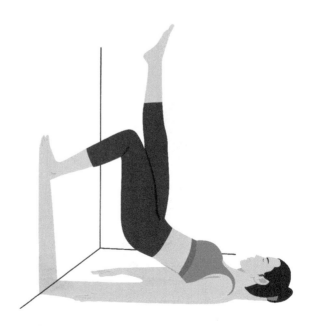

10.2 SINGLE LEG LIFT UPWARD HOLD

How: Similar to exercise 10.1, but instead of pulsing with one straight leg, hold it in the extended position for 10 counts.

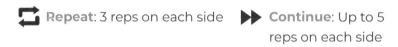 **Repeat**: 3 reps on each side   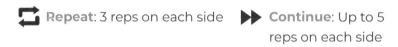 **Continue**: Up to 5 reps on each side

Modification: You may bend the knee on the extended leg if there are hamstring limitations.

Important notes: Keep the hips at the same height and active the glutes during the hold. Maintain your breathing during the hold.

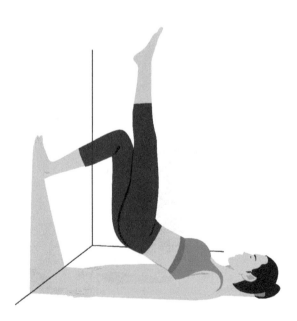

10.3 SINGLE LEG LIFT SIDEWAYS MOVEMENTS

How: Return to the single leg lift with the hip lift exercise. With one foot remaining against the wall to help to stabilize the body, lift and extend one leg and move it sideways. Return to the center in a slow and controlled movement.

 Repeat: 10 reps on each side   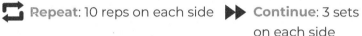 **Continue**: 3 sets on each side

Modification: You may bend the knee on the extended leg if there are hamstring limitations.

Important notes: Maintain the hips at the same height, squeeze the glutes to protect your lower back, and do not place any pressure on the back of the neck.

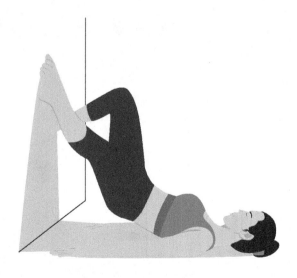

CHALLENGE DAY

11

SIT-UPS

11.1 BENT KNEES SIT-UPS (ARMS HUGGING THE TREE UNDER THE HAMSTRINGS)

How: Lower yourself to the floor. Bring your hips to the wall and bend your knees with both feet flat and about hip distance apart against the wall. Keep the knees at a 90-degree angle with your back and the back of your head on the floor. Imprint your lower back on the floor to protect your lower back. Lift your head from the ground as you tuck your chin to your chest. To protect your neck, leave a small space the size of an orange or tennis ball between the chin and chest. Engage your core to lift your upper back and mid back from the ground. Round your arms behind your hamstrings as you sit up. Hold that position for 3 counts before you slowly lower back down to the floor.

 Repeat: 20 reps   **Continue**: 3 sets

Modification: No holds during the sit-ups.

Important notes: Contract the ab muscles to maximize the effect. Be mindful of your neck position during the sit-ups.

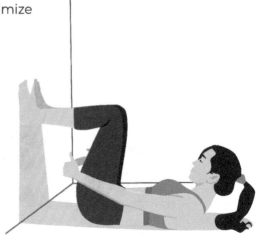

11.2 SPLIT LEGS SIT-UPS

How: Similar to exercise 11.1, but this time with legs extended to the sides. Split and stretch the legs away from each other, point or flex the toes, engage your core, and lift yourself upwards towards the wall with your arms reaching forward to walk your fingertips on the wall. Hold here for 3 counts before you slowly lower back down to the floor.

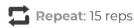 **Repeat**: 15 reps   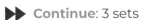 **Continue**: 3 sets

> **Modification**: Maintain a slight bend on your knees if your hamstrings are feeling tight. Avoid holds if you are not ready.

> **Important notes**: Contract the ab muscles to maximize the effect. Tuck the chin to the chest and leave an orange or tennis ball-sized space between the chin and chest to protect your neck.

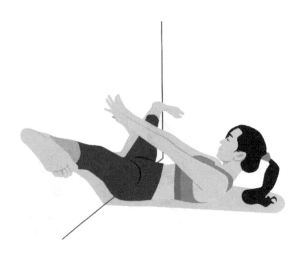

11.3 EXTENDED DOUBLE LEGS & EXTENDED OBLIQUES CRUNCH

How: Keep your hips towards the wall and extend both legs against the wall. Keep your back and the back of your head flat on the floor. Slowly lift your head and tuck your chin to your chest, leaving a small space the size of an orange or tennis ball between the chin and chest to protect your neck. Lift your arms and interlace your fingers, extending the 2 index fingers to point towards your right side, targeting the right oblique crunch. Continue crunching on this side of the obliques before lowering back down slowly and switching sides.

 Repeat: 20 reps   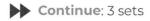 **Continue**: 3 sets

Modification: Lower the number of reps and sets if needed.

Important notes: Engage the obliques during the crunches to maximize the effect. Keep a microbend in your knees to avoid locking them.

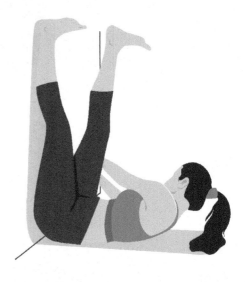

CHALLENGE DAY 12

12

LOWER BODY STRETCH & STRENGTHEN

12.1 SINGLE LEG STRETCH OUT AND STRENGTHEN

How: Lie down on the floor and bring your hips towards the wall. Extend both legs against the wall. Stretch one leg away and downwards, pointing your toes and using slow, controlled movement. The other leg remains stationary against the wall. Bring the leg back up to its starting position slowly. Complete the reps and sets before switching sides.

 Repeat: 20 reps on each side 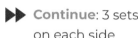 **Continue**: 3 sets on each side

Modification: Adjust the leg movement within a comfortable range of motion.

Important notes: Only one leg moves at a time. Maintain neutral hips throughout the exercise.

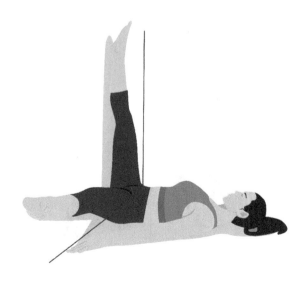

12.2 EXTENSION AND FLEXION KNEE PULSES

How: Lie down on the floor and bring your hips towards the wall. Extend both legs against the wall. Bend one knee and then extend the same leg. Continue this movement of extending and bending the knee to create downward and upward movement as if you are drawing the letter W. Repeat 10 reps on the same side, 3 sets each, before switching sides.

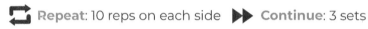 **Repeat**: 10 reps on each side   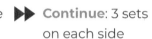 **Continue**: 3 sets on each side

Modification: Adjust the leg movement within a comfortable range of motion.

Important notes: Only one leg moves at a time. Maintain neutral hips throughout the exercise. Be mindful not to lock the knee.

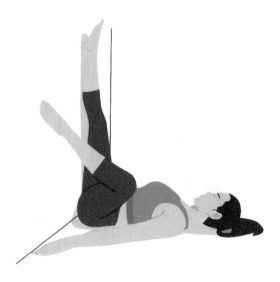

12.3 DOUBLE LEG STRETCH OUT AND STRENGTHEN

How: Lie down on the floor and bring your hips towards the wall. Extend both legs against the wall. Your back, the back of your head, and your arms are flat on the ground, with your arms next to your hips. Engage your core and glutes to protect your lower back. Flex both feet and stretch the legs away from each other slowly down to the floor. Now point the toes and activate the legs to draw them back together to their original position.

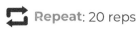 **Repeat**: 20 reps   ▶▶ **Continue**: 3 sets

Modification: Maintain a slight bend of your knees if your hamstrings are feeling tight.

Important notes: Flex the feet going down and point the toes going upwards. Don't move your back. The movement should be only in your legs.

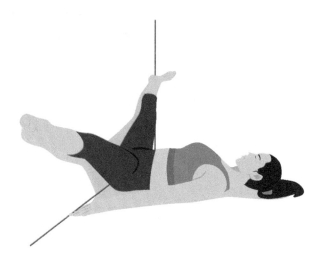

CHALLENGE DAY 13

CHAIR POSE

13.1 CHAIR POSE HOLD

How: Stand upright and bring your back against the wall. Lower your hips against the wall and walk the feet forward until the angle of the knees is 90 degrees. Hold the knees together with the toes pointing forward. Bring your hands to your hips and hold in this position for 30 seconds before slowly returning to upright against the wall.

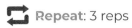 **Repeat**: 3 reps   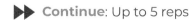 **Continue**: Up to 5 reps

Modification: Place your arms next to your hips and your palms on the wall.

Important notes: Squeeze your inner thighs and activate your glutes. Remove any pressure on your knee joints.

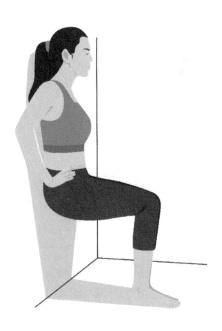

13.2 CHAIR POSE ALTERNATE HEEL RAISE

How: Similar to exercise 13.1, but instead of holding the pose, raise the heels one by one, alternating for 30 seconds before bringing yourself slowly back to upright against the wall.

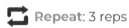 **Repeat**: 3 reps   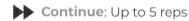 **Continue**: Up to 5 reps

Modification: Place your arms next to your hips and your palms on the wall.

Important notes: Ensure the heel is fully lifted and use the ball of the foot to balance.

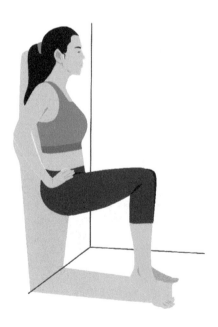

13.3 CHAIR POSE DOUBLE HEELS RAISE

How: Similar to exercise 13.2, but instead of a single heel raise, lift both heels for 5 counts before returning them to the floor. Continue this movement for 30 seconds on each rep.

 Repeat: 30 seconds   **Continue**: 3- 5 reps

Modification: Place your arms next to your hips and your palms on the wall.

Important notes: Ensure your heels are fully lifted and use the ball of the feet to balance.

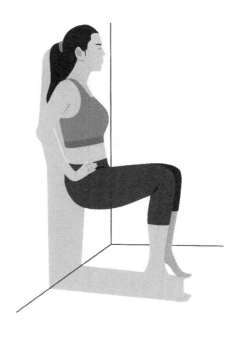

CHALLENGE DAY 14

14

HIGH PLANK
(palms on the ground)

14.1 HIGH PLANK HOLD

How: Bring your palms to the floor and spread your fingertips wide with the wrists under the shoulders. Extend and walk your feet against the wall until the hips and shoulders are at the same height. Protract your shoulder blades and engage your core. Hold here for 30 seconds while gazing down in between the thumbs. Slowly lower one knee to return safely to starting position.

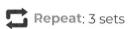 **Repeat**: 3 sets   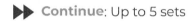 **Continue**: Up to 5 sets

Modification: Perform an elbow plank, similar to the high plank but with the elbows on the ground under the shoulders. Lower your feet if you find there's too much tension on the shoulder joints.

Important notes: Keep the core engaged and squeeze the glutes to protect your lower back.

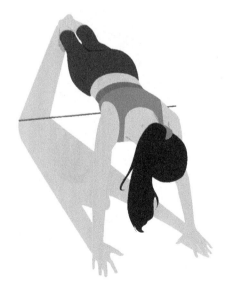

14.2 HIGH PLANK SINGLE LEG LIFTS WITH UPWARD PULSES

How: Start in the position of exercise 14.1, but as you stabilize in your high plank, slowly lift one leg upward without compromising your lower back and core engagement. Point or flex that lifted foot. Lower the foot against the wall. Repeat 10 reps on each side before switching sides.

 Repeat: 10 reps   **Continue**: 3 sets

Modification: Perform an elbow plank, similar to a high plank but with the elbows under the shoulders instead of the hands.

Important notes: Keep the core engaged to avoid lower back discomfort.

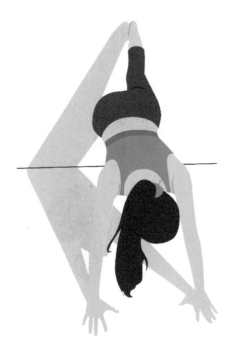

14.3 HIGH PLANK SINGLE LEG LIFTS WITH SIDEWAYS TOE TAP

How: Start in the position of exercise 14.1, but as you stabilize in your high plank, slowly lift one leg, move the leg to the side, and point the toes to tap down and up. Return to the starting position to complete 1 rep.

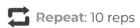 **Repeat**: 10 reps   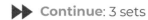 **Continue**: 3 sets

Modification: Perform an elbow plank, similar to a high plank but with the elbows under the shoulders instead of the hands.

Important notes: Keep the core engaged to avoid lower back discomfort.

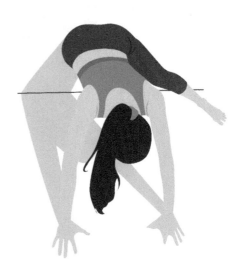

CHALLENGE DAY

15

SQUAT

15.1 SQUAT WITH CAT AND COW HIP MOVEMENTS

How: Stand upright and bring your back against the wall. Lower your hips against the wall and walk your feet outwards to form a squat. Keep the knees and toes pointing in the same direction. Bring your hands to your hips. Gently tilt and tuck your hips to perform a cat and cow hip movement by inhaling and tilting your tailbone, then exhaling and tucking your tailbone. Continue this movement for 30 seconds before slowly returning to starting position.

 Repeat: 3 reps   **Continue**: Up to 5 reps

Modification: Keep the hips higher if lowering the hips seems more challenging. Place your arms next to your hips and your palms on the wall.

Important notes: Maintain core engagement and avoid overcurving the lumbar, especially during cow movement (tilting the tailbone).

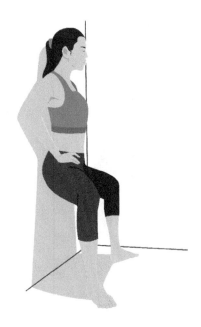

15.2 SQUAT WITH A HIP THRUST FORWARD

How: Stand upright and bring your back against the wall. Lower your hips against the wall and walk your feet outwards to form a squat. Bring your hands to your hips. Engage your core, squeeze your glutes, push your hips forward, and then return to the original position. Continue with this movement for 30 seconds before bringing yourself back up against the wall slowly.

 Repeat: 3 sets **Continue**: Up to 5 sets

Modification: Keep the hips higher if lowering the hips seems more challenging. Place your arms next to your hips and your palms on the wall.

Important notes: Maintain core engagement and avoid overcurving the lumbar.

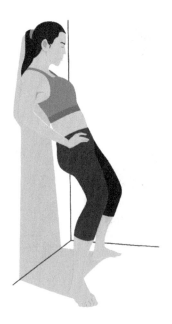

15.3 WIDE SQUAT PULSES

How: Stand upright and bring your back against the wall. Bring your hands to your hips. Walk the feet outwards to form a wider squat. Engage your core, squeeze your glutes, and drop your hips low as you bend your knees, then push back up to the original position with your feet and strong active legs. Continue with this movement, performing downward and upward pulses according to the reps and sets.

 Repeat: 15 reps   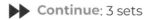 **Continue**: 3 sets

Modification: Place your arms next to your hips and your palms on the wall.

Important notes: Keep the pulses slow and controlled. Keep the knees and toes tracking in the same direction.

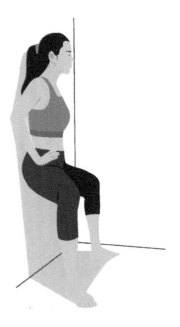

CHALLENGE DAY

16

BIRD DOG

(palms on the wall)

16.1 BIRD DOG HOLD AND STRETCH

How: Starting from the floor, face the wall and place the palms against the wall. Push against the palms to elongate your spine and bring the knees under your hips. Keep shoulders and hips at the same height. Extend one leg and lift it away from the ground, making sure the leg extension is at the same height as your hips and shoulder. Stay in this hold for 30 seconds before lowering the leg down to the floor slowly.

 Repeat: 3 sets   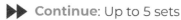 **Continue**: Up to 5 sets

Modification: Extend one leg with the toes on the ground.

Important notes: Maintain core engagement and avoid over-curving the lumbar.

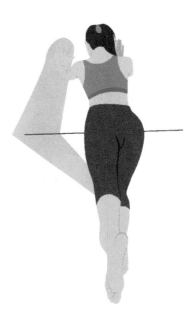

16.2 BIRD DOG EXTENDED LEG WITH ALTERNATE FOOT FLEXION AND EXTENSION PULSES

How: Similar to exercise 16.1, but instead of holding the pose, lift the extended leg and pulse it while alternately flexing and pointing the same foot. Continue this movement for 30 seconds.

 Repeat: 3 sets   **Continue**: Up to 5 sets

Modification: Extend one leg with the toes on the ground.

Important notes: Maintain core engagement and avoid over-curving the lumbar.

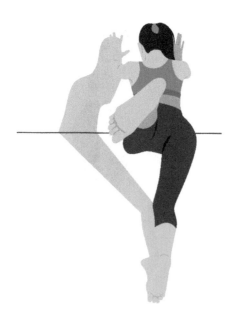

16.3 BIRD DOG EXTENDED LEG ROTATIONS

How: Similar to exercise 16.2, but instead of pulsing the extended leg, externally rotate the leg 15 times, and then internally rotate the leg 15 times, before slowly lowering the leg back to the floor.

Repeat: 2 sets on each side   **Continue**: Up to 5 sets on each side

Modification: Extend one leg with the toes on the ground and draw the rotations with your big toe.

Important notes: Maintain core engagement and avoid over-curving the lumbar.

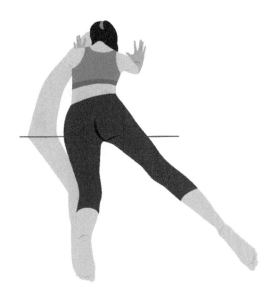

CHALLENGE DAY 17

17

THREAD THE NEEDLE

17.1 SUPPORTED THREAD THE NEEDLE STRETCH

How: Starting from the floor, face the wall and place the palms against the wall. Push against the palms to elongate your spine and bring the knees under your hips.

Lift one arm, reach up without moving the hips, and lower the same arm down and under the opposite arm to obtain the thread the needle pose. Hold in this pose for 30 seconds before switching sides.

Repeat: 1 set on each side   **Continue**: Up to 3 sets on each side

Modification: The reach of the arm under the arm on the wall can stay high if there are back limitations.

Important notes: Try your best not to move the hips during the spinal rotation.

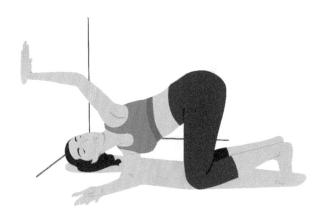

17.2 SPINAL EXTENSION AND FLEXION

How: Similar to exercise 17.1, start from the floor and face the wall, with the palms against the wall. Push against the palms to elongate your spine and bring your knees under your hips. Tuck your toes if this helps you stabilize. Lift your head and stretch forward to extend your spine without changing the original position of the hips and knees. Tuck your tailbone, flex your spine (curve your spine), and tuck your chin to your chest without changing the original position of the hips and knees.

 Repeat: 10 reps **Continue**: Up to 15 reps

Modification: Move the palms higher on the wall to make the movement more accessible for you.

Important notes: Move slowly as you articulate and control the spinal movement.

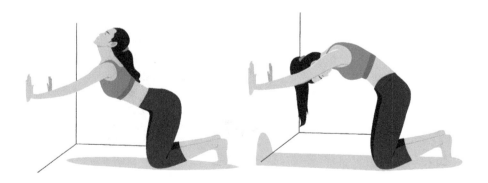

17.3 KNEELING ONE ELBOW TO FULL ARM PUSH-UPS WITH ONE ARM

How: Similar to exercise 17.1, start from the floor and face the wall at fingertips' distance from the wall. Bring the knees under your hips. Bend one arm to bring the elbow close to the wall and extend the other arm to the side. Maintain straight back alignment while pushing against the wall to perform a push up movement.

 Repeat: 15 reps   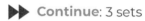 **Continue**: 3 sets

Modification: Move the palms higher on the wall to make the movement more accessible for you.

Important notes: Maintain core engagement and avoid over-curving the lumbar.

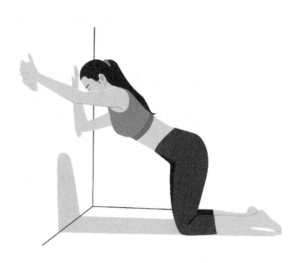

CHALLENGE DAY 18

HIP FLEXOR EXERCISES WITH EXTENDED LEG

18.1 HIP FLEXOR SINGLE LEG LIFT

How: Lower yourself to the floor with your back against the wall and extend both legs next to each other. Keep your hips neutral, your back flat on the wall, and both sit bones grounded. Place your arms on your sides with your fingertips touching the ground. Engage your core. Lift one leg, flex the foot, and maintain this hold for 5- 10 seconds. Slowly lower the leg.

 Repeat: 10 reps on each side ▶▶ **Continue**: 3 sets on each side

Modification: Place your hands on the sides of your hips and hold your palms down to the floor to assist with this exercise. Adjust the holding duration according to your capability.

Important notes: Maintain neutral hips and a straight back against the wall.

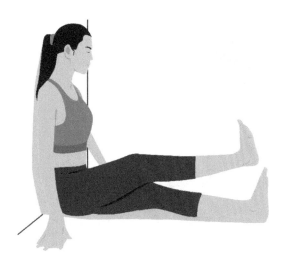

18.2 HIP FLEXOR SINGLE LEG CROSS

How: Similar to exercise 18.1, lower yourself to the floor with your back against the wall and extend both legs next to each other. Keep your hips neutral with your back flat on the wall and both sit bones grounded. Place your arms on your sides with your fingertips touching the ground. Engage your core. Lift one leg, flex the foot, and cross it over the opposite leg before returning it to its original position.

 Repeat: 15 reps on each side 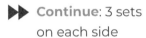 **Continue**: 3 sets on each side

Modification: Place your hands on the sides of your hips and hold your palms down to the floor to assist with this exercise.

Important notes: Maintain neutral hips and a straight back against the wall.

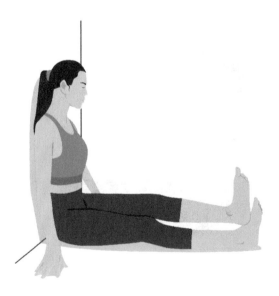

18.3 HIP FLEXOR SINGLE LEG SIDEWAYS

How: Similar to exercise 18.2, lower yourself to the floor with your back against the wall and extend both legs next to each other. Keep your hips neutral, your back flat on the wall, and both sit bones

grounded. Place your arms at your sides with your fingertips touching the ground. Engage your core. Lift one leg, flex the foot, and move the leg outwards before returning it to its original position. The other leg stays still and anchors to the floor during this movement.

 Repeat: 15 reps on each side   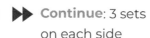 **Continue**: 3 sets on each side

Modification: Place your hands beside your hips and hold your palms down to the floor to assist with this exercise.

Important notes: Maintain neutral hips and a straight back against the wall.

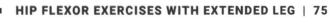

CHALLENGE DAY 19

19

SIDE PLANK

19.1 SIDE PLANK HOLD

How: Start on the floor, lying sideways with your back against the wall. Push your palm onto the ground, with the fingertips facing away from the wall. Lift yourself from the ground. Extend both legs against the wall. Keep the upper foot stacked onto the bottom foot or bring the upper foot in front of the bottom foot. Lift the upper arm and hold it against the wall to maintain this pose. Stay here for 30 seconds.

 Repeat: 3 sets on each side   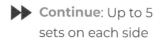 **Continue**: Up to 5 sets on each side

Modification: Instead of a full plank, lower one elbow down to perform an elbow plank. Instead of extending both legs, bend the upper knee as a support.

Important notes: Maintain core engagement and avoid over-curving the lumbar. Keep the chest lifted and engage the arm muscle for continuous support. Keep a microbend in the elbow to avoid hyperextending it.

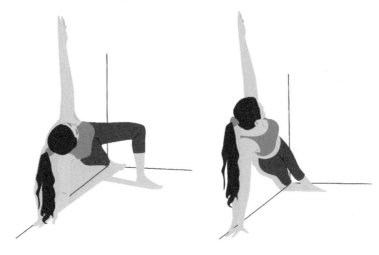

19.2 SIDE PLANK SINGLE LEG LIFT HOLD

How: Similar to exercise 19.1, but instead of lifting on both legs and holding the pose, lift the upper leg upwards, point the toes to activate the leg, and hold the position for 30 seconds.

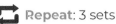 **Repeat**: 3 sets on each side   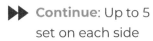 **Continue**: Up to 5 set on each side

Modification: Instead of a full plank, lower one elbow down to perform an elbow plank. Instead of extending both legs, bend the upper knee and bring it forward as a support. It is best to keep the upper heel against the wall for support during the hold.

Important notes: Maintain core engagement and avoid over-curving the lumbar. The upper leg remains active. Keep the chest lifted and engage the arm muscle for continuous support. Keep a microbend in the elbow to avoid hyperextending it.

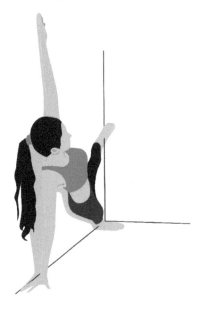

19.3 SIDE PLANK LEG LIFT TOE TAP FORWARD WITH EXTENDED LEG

How: Similar to exercise 19.1, but instead of holding the pose, adjust the position of the lower leg to 45 degrees forward for support. Lift the upper extended leg and drop it forward to perform a toe tap. Keep the hips neutral and engage the core during these movements.

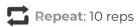 **Repeat**: 10 reps   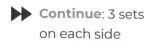 **Continue**: 3 sets on each side

Modification: Instead of a full plank, lower one elbow down to perform an elbow plank. Instead of extending both legs, bend the upper knee as a support. If extending the upper leg forward limits your movement, bend the upper knee forward and toe tap slowly.

Important notes: Maintain core engagement and avoid overcurving the lumbar. The upper leg remains active. Keep the chest lifted and engage the arm muscle for continuous support.

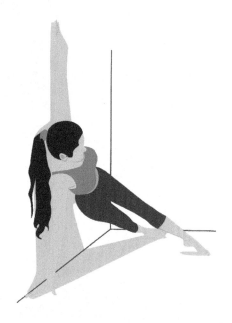

CHALLENGE DAY 20

BIRD DOG

(palms on the wall)

20.1 BIRD DOG EXTENDED LEG RAINBOW

How: Start by kneeling in front of the wall. Press against the wall with your palms as you adjust the knees under the hip position. Extend one leg out and flex that foot. Maintain hip neutrality. Engage your core and shoulder blade protraction. Bring the extended leg over to the outer side of the opposite foot to rainbow tap, making the arc shape of a rainbow between the first and second taps.

 Repeat: 15 reps   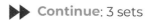 **Continue**: 3 sets

Modification: Bend the knee instead of extending the other leg. Take that knee behind the opposite knee to tap instead.

Important notes: Monitor your hip movement.

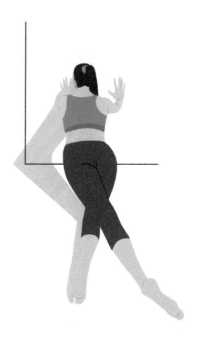

20.2 BIRD DOG EXTENDED LEG UPWARD PULSES

How: Similar to exercise 20.1, except extend one leg, keep it flexed or pointed, and pulse the leg upwards slowly and with control. Activate your glutes.

 Repeat: 15 reps   **Continue**: 3 sets

Modification: Bend the knee instead of extending the leg and pulse it upwards.

Important notes: Monitor your hip movement, keeping it neutral during the pulses.

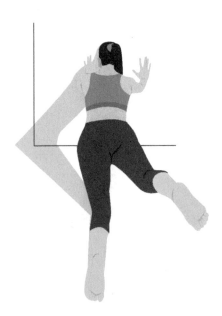

20.3 **BIRD DOG EXTENDED LEG SIDEWAYS**

How: Similar to exercise 20.1, but once you lift the extended leg with flexed or pointed toes, take it sideways and then return to the original position. During this movement, keep your glutes active.

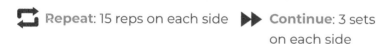 **Repeat**: 15 reps on each side ▶▶ **Continue**: 3 sets on each side

Modification: Bend the knee instead of extending the leg and move it sideways.

Important notes: Maintain control, as moving the leg or knee sideways may compromise your core engagement.

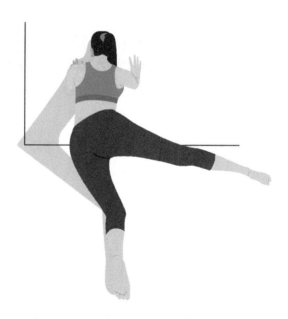

CHALLENGE DAY 21

21

SIDE-LYING

21.1 ADDUCTOR STRETCH WITH ONE BENT KNEE HOLD

How: Lie on the side of the wall with your back against the wall. Rest the side of your temple on the ground with the arm extended under your ear and the upper palm on the ground for support. Bend the bottom knee for additional support. Lift the upper extended leg high to stretch your inner thighs, holding that position for 30 seconds. Keep that leg active by pointing or flexing the foot.

 Repeat: 1 rep on each side   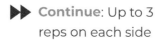 **Continue**: Up to 3 reps on each side

Modification: Bend the upper knee instead of extending it.

Important notes: Your back remains against the wall for support.

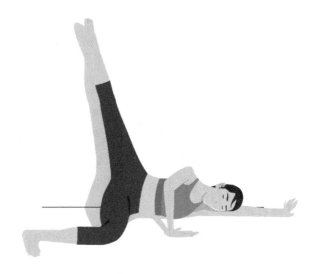

21.2 SINGLE LEG DROP FORWARD

How: Similar to exercise 21.1, as you lift one extended leg, bring that leg forward, lower it down to the floor, tap the pointed toes, and return to the starting position.

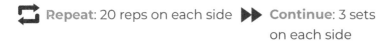 **Repeat**: 20 reps on each side 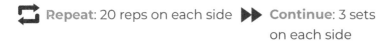 **Continue**: 3 sets on each side

Modification: Bend the upper knee instead of extending it, and kick the knee forward and return to starting position.

Important notes: Your back remains against the wall for support.

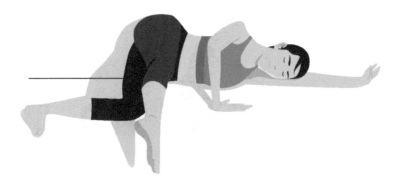

21.3 BENT KNEES CLAM PULSES

How: Similar to exercise 21.1, but with both knees bent at 45-degree angles. Bring the knees, heels, and toes on top of each other in the starting position. Ensure the head, shoulders, hips, heels, and toes are in the same alignment. Lift the upper knee away from the bottom knee without changing the position of the heels and toes. Return to the original position.

 Repeat: 20 reps on each side ▶▶ **Continue**: 3 sets on each side

Modification: If you're unable to reach the upper knee towards the wall, try to keep it lifted away from the bottom knee during the movements before slowly lowering it back down.

Important notes: Your back remains against the wall for support. Keep the inner thighs (adductors) active during this exercise.

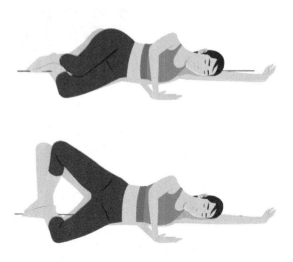

CHALLENGE DAY

22

LEG
WALK

22.1 WALK UPWARDS AND DOWNWARDS

How: Get into preparation for a hip lift with the feet pressed firmly against the wall. Activate the glutes and engage the core. Lift one foot and then the other, and walk upwards and downwards against the wall. Continue for 45 seconds. Lower your hips slowly to return to starting position.

 Repeat: 45 seconds   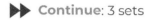 **Continue**: 3 sets

Modification: Leave the hips on the floor as you walk the feet upwards and downward slowly with control.

Important notes: During the hip lift and walking motion, keep the core engaged and the hips at the same height.

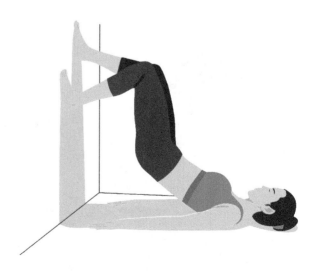

22.2 BUTTERFLY BRIDGE HIP THRUST

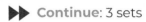

How: Get into preparation for a hip lift. Press the bottom feet together against the wall and bring the knees about shoulder-width distance apart. Place your palms down on the floor with the arms on the sides of your hips for support. Push your hips upwards by squeezing the glutes and inner thighs, then slowly lower the hips. Continue for 45 seconds for 1 set.

Repeat: 45 seconds   **Continue**: 3 sets

Modification: You can lower the hip position to make the movement more accessible.

Important notes: Maintain core engagement to avoid overcurving the lumbar.

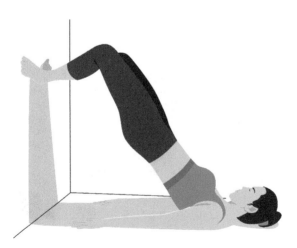

22.3 DOUBLE EXTENDED ALTERNATE SINGLE-KNEE PULSES

How: Get into preparation for a hip lift. Extend both legs upwards against the wall with a 45-degree angle, and keep the hips lifted. Place your palms down on the floor with the arms extended to the side of the hips for support. Bend one knee and draw it closer to your chest in pulses. Continue by extending that leg to complete the movement. Do this for 30 seconds before switching to the opposite side.

 Repeat: 30 seconds on each sides

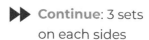 **Continue**: 3 sets on each sides

Modification: Instead of lifting the hips, keep the hips on the ground.

Important notes: Maintain core engagement to avoid overcurving the lumbar.

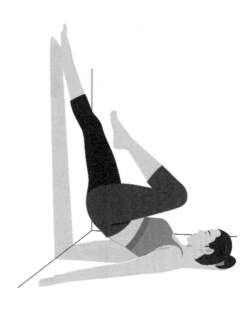

CHALLENGE DAY

23

**BEAR
PLANK**

23.1 BEAR PLANK HOLD

How: Bring yourself to a kneeling position on the ground facing the wall. Adjust your position, placing the knees underneath your hips about hips' distance apart. You may choose to tuck or untuck your toes. Keep the spine long and your palms against the wall around shoulder height. Look down to the floor so your neck extends at the same level as your spine. Inhale and lift your knees from the ground. Maintain this for 15-30 seconds. Slowly drop the knees one at a time.

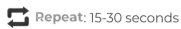 **Repeat**: 15-30 seconds   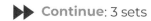 **Continue**: 3 sets

Modification: You may shorten the hold and continue with the knees on the ground.

Important notes: Keep your shoulders and hips on the same level. During the hold, maintain core engagement.

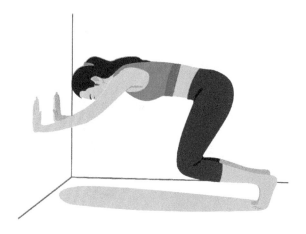

23.2 BEAR PLANK ALTERNATE KNEE TAPS

How: Similar to exercise 23.1, but instead of holding the pose, tap one knee and then switch to the other knee within 15-30 seconds. Slowly drop the knees one at a time to complete 1 set.

 Repeat: 15-30 seconds   **Continue**: 3 sets

Modification: You may shorten the duration of the hold and continue alternate knee tapping when you're ready.

Important notes: Keep your shoulders and hips at the same level. Maintain your hips at the same height during the alternate knee taps.

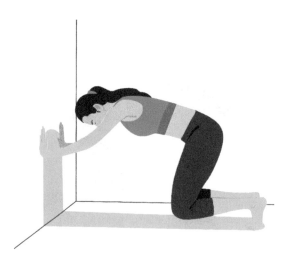

23.3 BEAR PLANK ALTERNATE KNEE CRISS-CROSS

How: Similar to exercise 23.1, but instead of holding the pose, draw one knee to the opposite side of the body, then switch knees and do the same. Continue for 15-30 seconds to complete 1 set.

 Repeat: 15-30 seconds   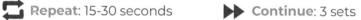 **Continue**: 3 sets

Modification: You may shorten the duration of the hold and continue alternate knee crisscrossing when you're ready.

Important notes: Warm up your wrists and toes. Keep the hip and shoulders at the same level during the movements by engaging your core and glutes.

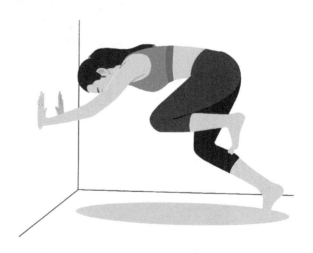

24

SWAN
DIVE

24.1 BABY SWAN DIVE

How: Lie down on the floor in a prone position. Face the wall and bring both elbows next to your ribcage. Place your palms against the wall. Keep your legs extended with the toes pointed to activate them. Activate your glutes to protect your lower back. Inhale and push your elbows down and your palms against the wall to lift your chest. Elongate your spine during this stretch. Exhale and slowly lower yourself back down to complete 1 rep.

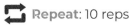 **Repeat**: 10 reps   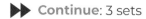 **Continue**: 3 sets

Modification: Control the chest lift during this stretch according to your flexibility.

Important notes: Avoid lower back discomfort by activating your glutes and maintaining the elongation of your spine.

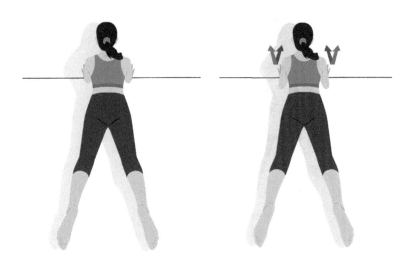

24.2 SWAN DIVE

How: Similar to the starting position in exercise 24.1, but instead of bending the elbows next to the ribcage, extend both arms upwards with the palms touching the wall. Inhale and push your elbows down and your palms against the wall to lift your chest. Elongate your spine during this stretch. Exhale and slowly lower yourself back down for 1 rep.

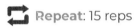 **Repeat**: 15 reps   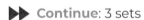 **Continue**: 3 sets

Modification: Adjust the chest lift during this stretch according to your flexibility.

Important notes: Avoid lower back discomfort by activating your glutes and maintaining the elongation of your spine.

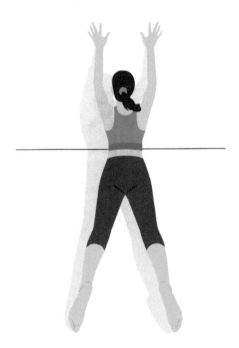

24.3 SWAN DIVE TWIST

How: Similar to exercise 24.2, but extend one arm upwards with the palm against the wall while the other arm is in an external rotation. Turn sideways and behind you to form a twist, turning your gaze to your hand and forming a fist with a thumbs up. Slowly return to the starting position and repeat the twist movement on the same side for 15 reps before switching sides.

 Repeat: 15 reps on each side   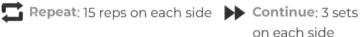 **Continue**: 3 sets on each side

Modification: Adjust the chest lift during this stretch according to your flexibility. Perform the spinal twist according to your range of motion.

Important notes: Avoid lower back discomfort by activating your glutes and maintaining the elongation of your spine. Ensure the stabilizing palm against the wall is pressing during the twist.

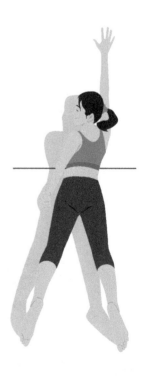

25

CAMEL (HIP) THRUST TO CHILD STRETCH

25.1 KNEES TOGETHER

How: Face the wall in a kneeling position with the knees together and the hips neutral. Choose to tuck or untuck your toes. Place your fingertips on your hips. Inhale, lift your chest upwards as you perform a mild backbend, and push your hips towards the wall. Protect your lower back by activating your glutes and elongating your spine. Keep the chest lifted upwards and open the chest. Hold here for 5 seconds while maintaining normal breathing. Then inhale, slowly lift your chest upwards to come out of the pose, and place your fingertips on the wall for balance.

 Repeat: 10 reps   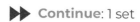 **Continue**: 1 set

Modification: Place your fingertips on the wall instead of the hips for additional support and balance.

Important notes: Once you complete one set, return to the child's pose as a counter pose to avoid lower back discomfort.

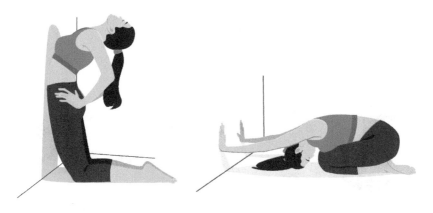

25.2 KNEES APART

How: Similar to exercise 25.1, but place the knees about hip distance apart with the heels together and the toes away from each other. Hold here for 5 seconds while maintaining normal breathing. Then inhale, slowly lift your chest upwards to come out of the pose, and place your fingertips on the wall for balance.

 Repeat: 10 reps   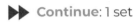 **Continue**: 1 set

Modification: Place your fingertips on the wall for additional support and balance.

Important notes: Once you complete one set, return to the child's pose as a counter pose to avoid lower back discomfort.

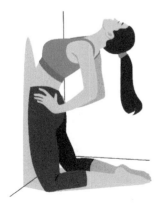
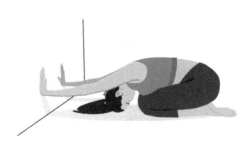

25.3 KNEES INWARD

How: Similar to exercise 25.1, but turn the knees inwards (internal rotation) to face each other with the heels and toes away from each other. Hold here for 5 seconds while maintaining normal breathing. Then inhale, slowly lift your chest upwards to come out from the pose, and place your fingertips on the wall for balance.

 Repeat: 10 reps   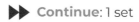 **Continue**: 1 set

Modification: Place your fingertips on the wall for additional support and balance.

Important notes: Once you complete one set, return to child's pose as a counter pose to avoid lower back discomfort.

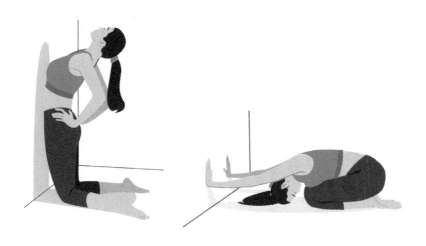

CHALLENGE DAY 26

26

CHAIR POSE

26.1 HOLD WITH ALTERNATE KNEE LIFT

How: Stand upright and bring your back against the wall. Lower your hips against the wall and walk the feet forward until the knees are at a 90-degree angle with the knees together and the toes pointing forward. Lift both arms above your knees. Lift one leg up and slowly drop it down gently to the ground. Continue on the opposite side, repeating for 30 seconds.

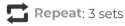 **Repeat**: 3 sets   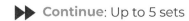 **Continue**: Up to 5 sets

Modification: Place your arms next to your hips and your palms on the wall.

Important notes: Squeeze your inner thighs and activate your glutes. Remove any pressure on your knee joints. Keep the hips on the same level and your back against the wall.

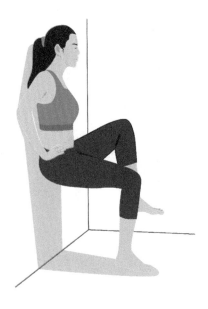

26.2 HOLD WITH SINGLE KNEE PULSES

How: Similar to exercise 26.1, but instead of alternating the knee lifts, lift one knee and pulse it upwards 15 times.

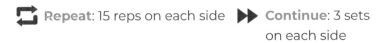 Repeat: 15 reps on each side   ▶▶ Continue: 3 sets
                                                              on each side

Modification: Place your arms next to your hips and your palms on the wall.

Important notes: Squeeze your inner thighs and activate your glutes. Remove any pressure on your knee joints. Keep the hips on the same level and your back against the wall.

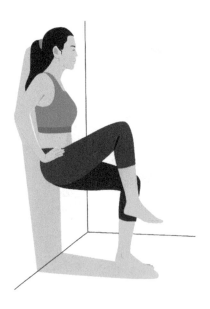

26.3 OBLIQUES ALTERNATE ELBOW / ARM REACH

How: Similar to exercise 26.1, but remain in your chair pose. Lift your arms upwards, interlace your fingers behind your head, and bend both elbows. Inhale and lengthen your spine. As you exhale, move one elbow down and sideways along the wall to stretch your lats and activate your obliques on the opposite side. Inhale and come back to the center. As you exhale, perform the same movement on the opposite side. Repeat in a controlled and slow manner for 30 seconds.

 Repeat: 3 sets   **Continue**: Up to 5 sets

Modification: Instead of interlacing your fingers behind your head, reach the fingertips downwards and to the side on the wall instead.

Important notes: Do not move your hips. Keep the knees together at all times, with the toes pointing forward in the same direction.

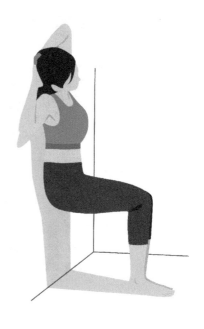

CHALLENGE DAY

27

SINGLE LEG STRETCH
(extended legs on the wall)
WITH HIPS ELEVATED

27.1 KNEE PULL AND EXTEND (SINGLE KNEE STRETCH)

How: Lie down on the floor and bring your hips close to the wall. Bend your knees and place your feet hip distance apart on the wall. Ensure the angle of the knees is 90 degrees, with your palms on the floor next to your hips. Press your palms firmly to the floor and engage your glutes, inner thighs, and core as you push through your upper back to lift your hips upwards, keeping the hips neutral. Walk both your legs up the wall until both legs are extended against the wall and the hips are elevated. Stabilize with your upper back and palms on the ground. Exhale, bend one knee, and pull it closer to your chest. Inhale and extend the leg. Repeat for 30 seconds before switching sides.

 Repeat: 3 sets on each side   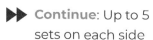 **Continue**: Up to 5 sets on each side

Modification: Instead of lifting the hips, ground your hips to the floor.

Important notes: Do not put any pressure on the back of your neck. Keep the hips the same level throughout the single knee stretch.

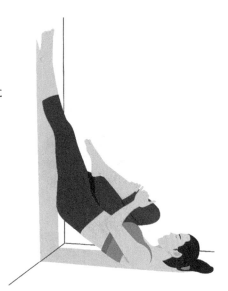

How: Lie down on the floor and bring your hips close to the wall. Bend your knees and place your feet hip distance apart against the wall. Ensure the angle of the knees is 90 degrees and your palms are on the floor next to your hips. Press your palms firmly, and engage your glutes, inner thighs, and core as you push through your upper back to lift your hips. Keep the hips neutral. Stabilize with your upper back and palms on the ground. Exhale and bend one knee to pull it closer to your chest, maintaining the knee angle 90 degrees with pointed toes. Hold for 30 seconds.

 Repeat: 3 sets on each side

 Continue: Up to 5 sets on each side

Modification: Instead of lifting the hips, ground your hips to the floor.

Important notes: Do not put any pressure on the back of your neck. Keep the hips at the same level throughout the single knee stretch.

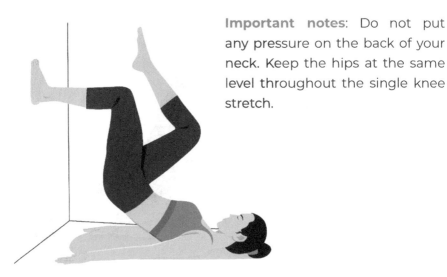

27.3 SINGLE-LEG SIDEWAYS STRETCH AND PULL

How: Similar to exercise 27.2, but instead of lifting one leg in a tabletop, extend one leg, point the toes to activate the leg, and bring the leg sideways (outer side) before slowly drawing it back to center. Repeat on the same side for 30 seconds.

 Repeat: 3 sets on each side   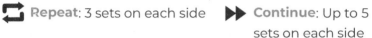 Continue: Up to 5 sets on each side

Modification: Instead of lifting the hips, ground your hips to the floor.

Important notes: Do not put any pressure on the back of your neck. Keep the hips at the same level throughout the single knee stretch. Stabilize through your upper back and with the foot that is against the wall.

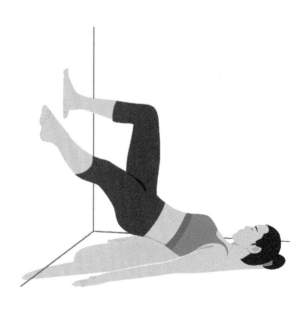

CHALLENGE DAY

28

NARROW
SQUAT

(with palms on the wall)

28.1 NARROW SQUAT PULSE

How: Stand facing the wall with the fingertips touching the wall and walk a few steps backwards. Lower the hips as you bring both knees together. Lift the heels off the ground and find your balance. Inhale, lift your hips, and as you exhale, drop your hips low into your narrow squat. Move in a pulsing movement for 30 seconds.

 Repeat: 3 sets   ▶▶ **Continue**: Up to 5 sets

Modification: Instead of lifting the heels off the ground, keep the feet flat on the ground in the starting position.

Important notes: Ensure your knees do not go beyond your toes to protect your knee joints. Keep your hips neutral and your core engaged during the movements.

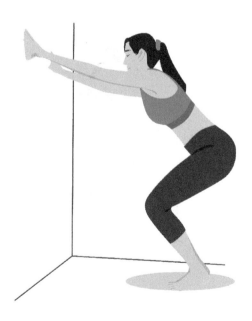

28.2 TRIPLE NARROW SQUAT PULSES WITH FIGURE FOUR KICKS

How: Similar to exercise 28.1, but instead of pulsing for 30 seconds, pulse only 3 times. Then lift your bent knee and point it outward at a 45 degree angle in a figure four. Kick it upwards for 1 rep. Point your toes when you're kicking upwards to activate your leg and (adductor) inner thigh. Continue these movements for 45 seconds on each side.

 Repeat: 3 sets on each side   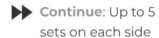 **Continue**: Up to 5 sets on each side

Modification: Lower the number of pulses depending on your capability.

Important notes: Ensure your knees do not go beyond your toes to protect your knee joints during the pulses. Keep your hips neutral and your core engaged during the movements.

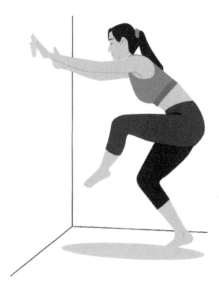

28.3 DEEP SQUAT WITH ALTERNATE SHOULDER DIPS AND HEEL RAISES

How: Stand facing the wall. From here, bring your palms against the wall and widen your stance by walking your feet outwards to form a wide squat. Engage your core, squeeze your glutes, and drop your hips low as you bend your knees. In your deep wide squat, drop one shoulder toward the ground and lift the heel on the same side. Then switch sides. Continue for 30 seconds.

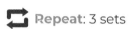 **Repeat**: 3 sets   ▶▶ **Continue**: Up to 5 sets

> **Modification**: Control the stretch during the shoulder dips according to your range of motion. Keep the feet flat instead of doing alternating heel raises.
>
> **Important notes**: As you lean your torso forward, be mindful of the pressure that you put on your knee joints.

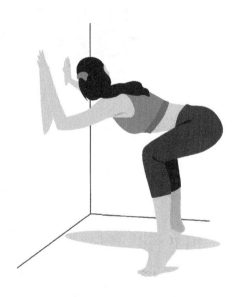

CHALLENGE DAY

29

BICYCLE

29.1 HIP LIFT BRIDGE SINGLE LEG EXTENSION UPWARDS AND TOE TAPS

How: Lie down on the floor and bring your hips close to the wall. Bend your knees and place your feet hip distance apart against the wall. Ensure the knee angle is 90 degrees and your palms are on the floor next to your hips. Press your palms down firmly and engage your glutes, inner thighs, and core as you push through your upper back to lift your hips. Keep the hips neutral. Lift one leg upwards with pointed toes, then bend the same knee and tap the pointed toes on the ground on the same side. Repeat 20 reps on the same side before switching sides.

 Repeat: 20 reps on each side 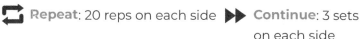 **Continue**: 3 sets on each side

Modification: Instead of lifting the hips, ground your hips to the floor.

Important notes: Do not put any pressure on the back of your neck when you perform the hip lift.

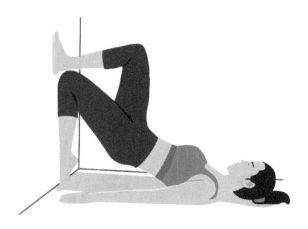

29.2 STRAIGHT-LEG SCISSORS

How: Get into preparation for a hip lift. Extend both legs upwards against the wall at a 45-degree angle. Place your arms on the sides of your hips, bend your elbows, and use your hands to support and lift your hips by pressing the elbows and upper shoulders against the ground. Lift one extended leg away from the ground, then bring it closer to you and switch legs. Continue alternating the extended legs in a scissor movements for 30 reps.

 Repeat: 30 reps   **Continue**: 3-5 sets

Modification: Lower your hips to the ground instead. Place your palms down on the floor with your arms at the sides of your hips for support.

Important notes: Do not put any pressure on the back of your neck when you perform the scissors movement in hip lift.

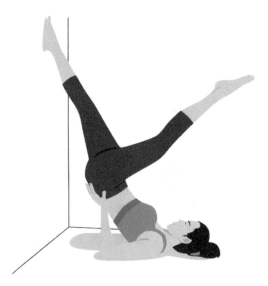

29.3 HIP-ELEVATED BICYCLES

How: Similar to exercise 29.2, but instead of extended legs, bend both knees at a 90-degree angle. Point the toes and elevate the hips with the support of your elbows and palms. Draw the knees closer to you one by one, alternating knees as if riding a bicycle. Repeat 30 times.

 Repeat: 30 reps   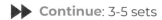 **Continue**: 3-5 sets

Modification: Lower your hips to the ground instead. Place your palms down on the floor with your arms on the sides of your hips for support.

Important notes: Do not put any pressure on the back of your neck when you perform the bicycle movement in hip lift. Elbows are close (turned in) to your body during the hip elevated exercise.

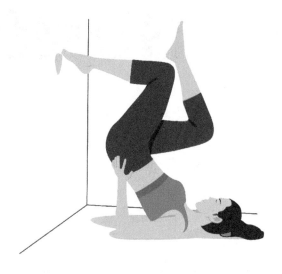

CHALLENGE DAY

30

THE
HUNDRED

30.1 THE HUNDRED IN TABLETOP

How: Lie down on the floor and bring your hips close to the wall. Bend your knees and place your feet hip distance apart on the wall. Ensure the angle of the knees is 90 degrees. Lift your arms slightly above the ground next to your hips. Engage your core and maintain a neutral hip. Lift your head, tuck your chin to your chest, and inhale for 5 counts while pulsing your arms up and down around the hip level. Then exhale for 5 counts, pulsing the arms to complete 10 reps. Continue for 100 reps in 1 set, then slowly return your mid back, upper back, and the back of your head to the ground and release your arms.

 Repeat: 100 reps   **Continue**: Just 1 set

Modification: Do lower reps depending on your ability, or rest in between the reps.

Important notes: Maintain core engagement and avoid over-curving the lumbar. Upper legs remain active. Keep the chest lifted and engage the arm muscles.

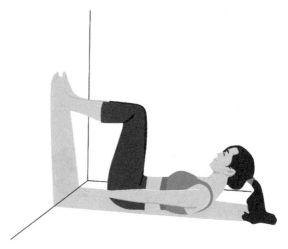

30.2 THE HUNDRED WITH 45-DEGREE DOUBLE LEG EXTENSION

How: Similar to exercise 30.1, but instead of legs in the table-top position of 90 degrees, extend the legs to the wall at a 45-degree angle.

 Repeat: 100 reps   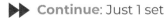 **Continue**: Just 1 set

Modification: Do lower reps depending on your ability, or rest in between the reps.

Important notes: Maintain core engagement and avoid over-curving the lumbar. Upper legs remain active. Keep the chest lifted and engage the arm muscles.

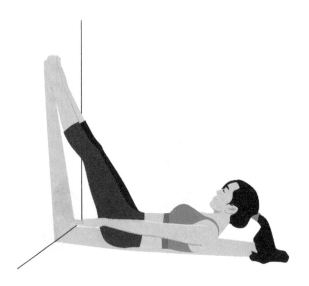

30.3 THE HUNDRED WITH 90-DEGREE DOUBLE LEG EXTENSION

How: Similar to exercise 30.1, but instead of positioning the legs in tabletop at 90 degrees, extend the legs upright against the wall.

 Repeat: 100 reps   **Continue**: Just 1 set

Modification: Do lower reps depending on your ability, or rest in between the reps.

Important notes: Maintain core engagement and imprint the lower back to the ground. The upper legs remain active. Point both toes. Squeeze the inner thighs. Keep the chest lifted and engage the arm muscles.

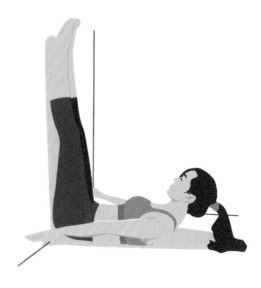

Made in the USA
Monee, IL
02 July 2024

61134138R00069